DEDICATION

I dedicate this book to my family. My family knows my strength and weakness and they are always there for me through thick and thin.

TABLE OF CONTENTS

Break Binge Eating

Be Healthy in No Time

By: Frederick Morgan

9781635013160

PUBLISHERS NOTES

Disclaimer – Speedy Publishing LLC

This publication is intended to provide helpful and informative material. It is not intended to diagnose, treat, cure, or prevent any health problem or condition, nor is intended to replace the advice of a physician. No action should be taken solely on the contents of this book. Always consult your physician or qualified health-care professional on any matters regarding your health and before adopting any suggestions in this book or drawing inferences from it.

The author and publisher specifically disclaim all responsibility for any liability, loss or risk, personal or otherwise, which is incurred as a consequence, directly or indirectly, from the use or application of any contents of this book.

Any and all product names referenced within this book are the trademarks of their respective owners. None of these owners have sponsored, authorized, endorsed, or approved this book.

Always read all information provided by the manufacturers' product labels before using their products. The author and publisher are not responsible for claims made by manufacturers.

This book was originally printed before 2014. This is an adapted reprint by Speedy Publishing LLC with newly updated content designed to help readers with much more accurate and timely information and data.

Speedy Publishing LLC

40 E Main Street, Newark, Delaware, 19711

Contact Us: 1-888-248-4521

Website: http://www.speedypublishing.co

REPRINTED Paperback Edition: ISBN: 9781635013160

Manufactured in the United States of America

Chapter 1- Introduction to a Fitter You

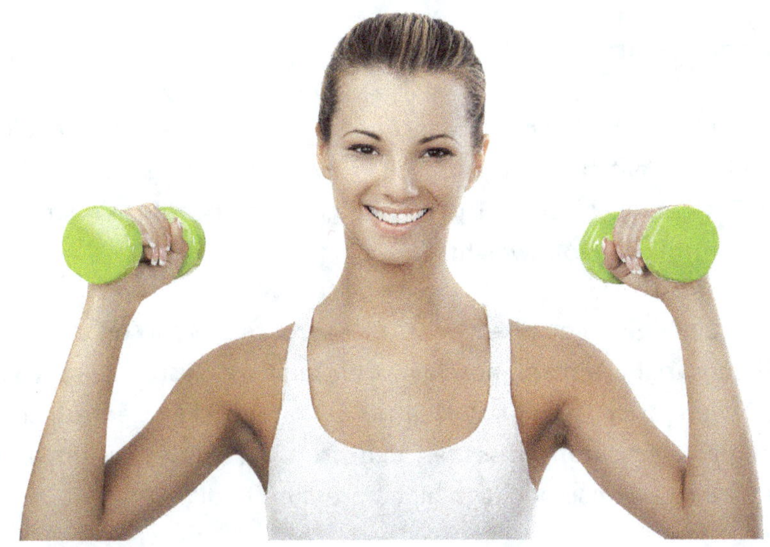

Sound eating isn't about rigid nutrition doctrines, staying unrealistically skinny, or depriving yourself of the foods you adore. As an alternative, it's about feeling excellent, having more energy, and keeping yourself as sound as possible- all of which might be attained by learning some nutrition basics and using them in a way that works for you.

Sound eating starts with learning how to "eat intelligently"-it's not simply what you eat, however how you eat. Your food choices might reduce your risk of illnesses like heart conditions, cancer, and diabetes, as well as battle against depression.

In addition, learning the habits of intelligent eating might boost your energy, heighten your memory and stabilize your mood. You are able to expand your range of sound food choices and learn how to plan ahead to produce and sustain a gratifying, intelligent diet. Get all the info you need here.

The Advantages

Let's straight-away launch into the subject.

You become fitter

We could have a whole collection of books about the health benefits of eating right and still it wouldn't quite cover what benefits genuinely exist. The most significant benefit is that you gain control over your weight.

By eating right, you likewise make sure that your metabolism functions right - most notably your immune system and your digestive system - keep working right. You are likewise protected from different chronic diseases, right from cardiovascular diseases like arterial sclerosis and high blood pressure to diabetes.

More cost-efficient

Eating healthy means you spend much less. Your bills at the supermarkets reduce drastically and you don't plunge farther into credit card debt if that's already an issue with you. In addition to that, you save a big bundle on all the healthcare expenses you'd need if any issue surfaces because of your food binging habits.

Fewer toxins within your body

Numerous foods nowadays are toxic because of the synthetic chemicals present in them. Once you are trying to eat right, you are much less likely to get these toxins into your body as one of the basic tenets of eating right is that you shouldn't eat anything that's man-made.

In addition to that, if you eat less, you will likewise be able to cut back on vices like smoking and alcoholism. A glass of beer is almost synonymous with a night out with the boys. If you eat less, you won't want the beer as well. Likewise, you will not want that one (or more) mandatory smoke that you tend to have after each meal.

More active life-style

Once you eat better, you will find that you're able to do your work in a much better way. You can exercise more, travel more, play more, work more and therefore make your life more productive.

That sure beats being a plump slob and lounging around on the couch the whole day, doesn't it? You're able to also be more involved with your friends and family and that surely enriches your life.

Great social life

Forget about fat fetishes, persons who are overweight don't look attractive. There's a strong social taboo about weight on the wrong places of the body. If you are trying to find a partner, your flab might virtually get in the way.

Not simply that, persons who can't control their eating habits and hence their weights are looked down on by society as being persons who can't control their basic urges.

This sort of psychology does exist, though very few persons will speak about it. Once you eat right, you will discover that such issues go away.

Break the Binge Habit

We have all been there: turning to the icebox if feeling lonely or bored or indulging in seconds or thirds if strained. But if you suffer from binge eating, the from time to time urge to overeat is more like an obsession.

Instead of eating sensibly to make up for it, you penalize yourself by purging, fasting, or exercising to do away with the calories.

You may have found how easily you're able to get rid of the food ingested during a "binge" by vomiting or taking diet pills or laxatives.

The vicious circle of binging and purging carries a toll for the body, and it's even harder on mental well-being. However the cycle might be broken.

Effective binge eating treatment and support might help you develop a healthier relationship with food and defeat feelings of tension, guilt, and shame. Binge eating nervosa is an eating disorder qualified by commonplace episodes of binge eating, followed by frantic efforts to avoid putting on weight.

If you're fighting with binge eating, life is a ceaseless battle between the want to slim down or remain thin and the overpowering obsession to binge eating.

You don't want to binge-you understand you'll feel guilty and ashamed subsequently-but over and over you succumb. During an average binge, you might devour from 3,000 to 5,000 calories in a single short hour.

After it stops, terror sets in and you turn to drastic measures to "undo" the binge, like taking ex-lax, inducing vomiting, or going on a ten-mile run. And all the time, you feel more and more out of control.

It's crucial to note that binge eating doesn't inescapably involve purging-physically doing away with the food from your body by barfing or utilizing laxatives, enemas, or diuretics. If you make up for your binges by fasting, working out to excess, or going on crash diets, this also qualifies as binge eating. If you're living with binge eating, you comprehend how scary it feels to be so out of command. Knowing that you're harming your body simply adds to the fear.

However buck up: change is possible. No matter how long you've fought with binge eating, you're able to learn to break the binge and purge cycle and develop a healthier attitude towards food and your body. Acknowledge you have an issue.

Up till now, you've been invested in the idea that life will be greater- that you'll at last feel good-if you drop off more weight and command what you eat. The first step in binge eating recovery is admitting that your relationship to food is garbled and out of command.

Talk to someone. It might be hard to discuss what you're going through, especially if you've kept your binge eating a secret for a while. You could be ashamed, ambivalent, or frightened of what others will think. However it's crucial to comprehend that you're not alone. Find a great listener-somebody who will support you as you attempt to get better.

Keep away from individuals, places, and activities that spark the temptation to binge or purge. You may need to avoid looking over fashion or fitness magazines, spend less time with friends that constantly diet and discuss losing weight, and stay away from weight loss sites and "pro-mia" sites that encourage binge eating.

You may likewise need to be careful when it comes to meal preparation and cooking magazines and shows. Seek professional help.

The advice and support of trained eating disorder pros might help you retrieve your health, learn to eat normally once more, and formulate healthier mental attitudes about food and your body.

CHAPTER 2- THE GLORY OF BINGE EATING ON NUTRITIOUS FOOD

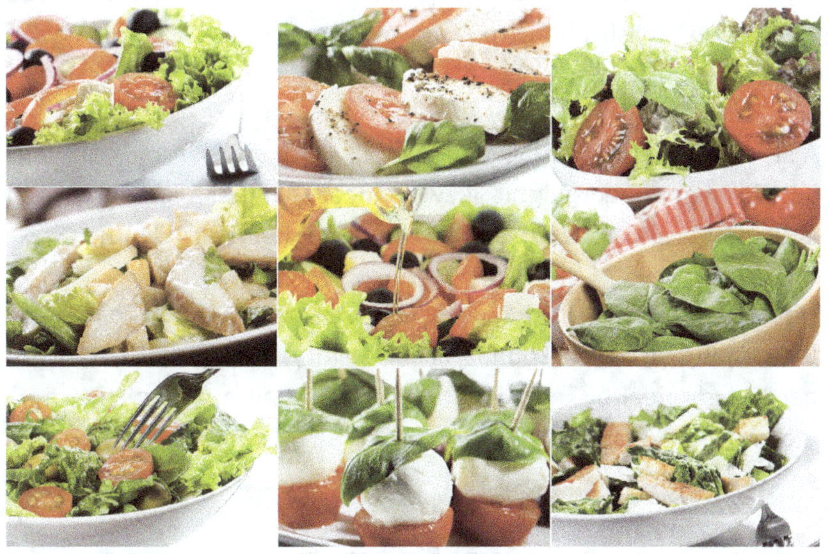

Cravings occur. Some of the times they seem to pop out of nowhere. Some of the times they're emotional. And some of the times they exist simply because I'm getting hungry! My feelings toward cravings have constantly been the same, regardless of the situation: I don't like them!

What we need is to seize a plan that will help in handling cravings the best way conceivable. In my experience, arriving at small shifts over time is simpler to adopt and is better than attempting to swap everything in one fell pounce.

I'm likewise sure that as I learn more, my fight plan might alter. The one I'll center on today is:

A select breakfast: The first step to combating cravings

Why breakfast? Breakfast presents the body fuel and keeps blood sugar levels steadier. I recognize that if I skip breakfast my blood glucose will crash about mid morning, and then I'll gorge myself silly come lunchtime.

A steadfast blood sugar level means I'll keep away from "crashing" and subsequent gorging. It likewise means I'll feel a lot alerter and industrious, and I need this as I'm not a morning individual!

Not all breakfasts are the equivalent, though. A mocha café latte with whipped cream sounds like a savory breakfast, but it's not particularly healthy, nor would it carry me all morning! If I say a "select" breakfast, I'm referring to a breakfast with a little protein and complex carbohydrates.

Complex carbohydrates carry fiber and more nutrients than the complicated stuff. Again, my blood sugar will be a lot less fluctuating, and that means I keep away from the sugar crash.

Protein will hold my hunger at bay for a longer time period.

Now the hard part: integrating all of this into a breakfast I'll really eat!

Here are a few breakfast selections I've come up with that I know I would love:

• Rich fiber, protein whole grain cereal with skim milk or soya milk

• Whole meal toast with scrambled eggs (made with for the most part egg whites)

• Oatmeal with a bit of protein powder, walnuts, and skimmed milk added to it (add don't forget chopped apples and cinnamon!)

• Breakfast burrito - scrambled eggs, veggies, low fat cheese in a whole grain tortilla

Food for the Soul

Some of the time people are so eager to try something new or the latest popular thing that they fail to realize that for anything to be a benefit, it have to first be understood and then utilized or practiced over a period of time.

Some of the time this time frame may take quite a while to show any noticeable results.

In the enthusiasm of it all, some might even overlook simple ways to having a better quality of life, being happier, healthier or merely just for healing. Meditation is one of these easy ways.

Meditation need not be a complicated procedure, nor need it be a religious process. All the same those who want to take the quest deeper might find spiritual fulfillment too. Naturally for meditation to work, it application and practice have to be right.

Being able to stay focused and centered throughout the meditative procedure is the key to reaping the benefits of meditation. The level of centeredness the individual has accomplished dictates his or her reactions and that of the surroundings.

Once there is a level of centeredness from inside the outer events adjust to the inner energy because the centered energy is solider than dissipated, reactive energy. Meditation is primarily the art of learning how to reach this level of centeredness. It is even referred to as the nearest link between one's spiritual nature and God.

Once the person does not understand the importance of attaining this centeredness, then the problems around, take on more significance. Resulting in the failure mentality seeping in and a lot of damaging energy is released.

Though we may never control all things especially outward influences, with the utilization of meditation it is possible to control our frame of mind and thus the reactive outcome. Meditation raises the level of consciousness and beefs up our aura.

Meditation is a tool. It might help combat stress, fosters physical health, aids with chronic pain, may make you sleep better, feel more pleased, be more peaceful, as well as be in the here and now. However on a deeper level, meditation is a door into the unknown. It may help us get a feel of the mystery of who we are.

Chapter 3- Mind Conditioning to Resist Unhealthy Diet

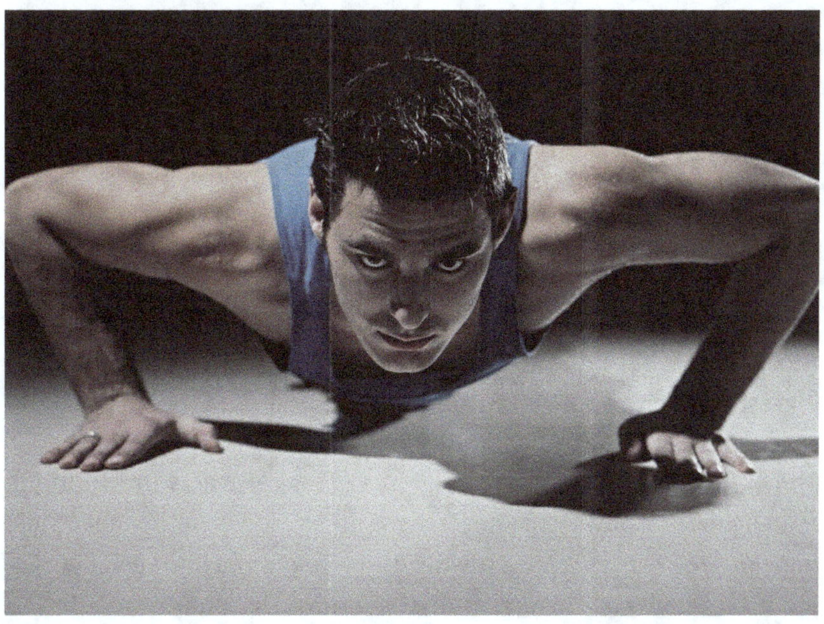

It's nearly impossible to have optimum living without the right type of mentality and tools. It doesn't matter what type of health you have now.

There's a particular way of thinking that you must have, and this type of thinking is what will give you the discipline to take action. Taking action is the most essential part of optimum living, and positive thoughts are called for to take major action.

If you're not ready with the right type of mentality then I fear you're destined to less than optimum living. Without the right type of mentality your health might fail. If you're considering how to achieve optimum living... you truly need this mentality and tools.

Affirmations are self-talk statements & better presented to the subconscious. These new images are viewed as "credible" by the subconscious & are placed in the area of subconscious having to do with the might to enhance the ability to pull up particular powerful memories with less work.

Through this particular imagery a person may develop the inner tools for the correct mentality for optimum living, letting the memories and images be transported to the present moment where they're used for enhancing mindset which is crucial for health and wellness.

Frequently individuals believe these good and beneficial self talk memories are a fallacy and don't exist, but the subconscious recognizes where they're located and will pull them ahead for increased health and wellness.

These forms of affirmations make new neural tracts in the mind, enhancing the power to "see" these fresh powerful images. Stale images related to negativeness, weaknesses, deficiency of initiative, frail goal images and the ability to acquire health and wellness plan are diminished. When the mind discovers new affirmations the subconscious mind sees them as "tangible."

You've likely observed a basic element in those who have achieved optimum living in business and in life. These winners and successful individuals tend to be enthusiastic and zealous, in all aspects of their lives. This exuberance may be infectious, and it tends to rub off on all those individuals around them. A positive mental attitude and the might to turn that mental attitude into results are essential to optimum living, both in business and life.

You see, a positive mental attitude is a valuable asset, regardless what your goals. You truly ought to assume the habit of doing regular favorable affirmations. Making positive affirmations a part of your daily function is a great way to alter your thoughts and help yourself acquire health and wellness.

It's never too early or too late to begin this cycle of favorable affirmations, and even those simply beginning down this path may benefit from a positive mental attitude. Even if your health seems poor and you're not yet living optimally, it's crucial to display a positive mental attitude, and not let negativity sneak in to steal your thunder.

Remember that some of the most successful individuals started somewhere. It truly is possible to attain optimum living, but without positive affirmations and a victorious mental attitude, this move won't be possible.

Steady positive affirmations are exceedingly crucial for those individuals who want optimum living. True health and wellness is never simple, but it's crucial to remember that those around you, from loved ones to clients to competitors, feel your mental attitude, and utilize it as a cue.

If you're perpetually complaining about the deficiency of well being, the individuals around you will be less than energized. If, on the other hand, you're perpetually supplying positive affirmations to yourself and the individuals around you, even in the hardest of times, they'll see your exuberance, learn from it, and use it as a cue to work harder and fix their own conditions.

It truly does all come down to mental attitude; a positive mental attitude and positive affirmations may help your health and wellness in ways too many to mention here.

Concoct ways to be physically active. Most heavy individuals spend much time considering what they're going to eat. Ideas of what snacks, lunches and suppers they're going to enjoy and once, are what outlines their schedule for the day.

In order to bear a successful mentality for weight loss, you have to start including ideas of physical activities with thoughts of food.

Physical action works best once it's a firm part of your life, and exercise at home might be much handier than attempting to find time to get to the gymnasium.

Moreover, exercise is commonly more gratifying if it takes place in a comfortable environment, and doing it at home provides you the ability to tailor the experience to fit your individual tastes.

If you're able to find easy, flexible strategies to add a little physical action into your routine, you'll stick with it more readily (and move on to more formal physical exertion more quickly).

A lot of us are hooked on our cars, however with simply a little shift; we might turn daily errands into a simple way to exercise. Instead of driving to the corner grocery, walk or ride a bicycle.

Purchase a cart to carry your supplies or a trailer to pull behind the bicycle. Any little neighborhood errands might be achieved in this manner.

Take the stairs instead of the elevator in your apartment house.

If you've youngsters, walk with them once you take excursions, instead of packing everybody into the car. A leisurely stroll to the local park gets everybody some fresh air while helping you feel great.

A sneaky way to fit physical action in is to do a little multitasking. Get a hands-free telephone system and utilize hand weights or do push- ups while you're waiting for the other person to pick up the telephone.

Discover tasks that entail standing (like vacuuming or dusting), and plan to engage in them a couple of times every day. Utilize ankle weights and take little "walking breaks" to stretch out your legs if you are able to.

Do 5 or 10 push-ups each time you enter or leave a room---nothing too long, simply a few seconds to get your motor running.

Make fun out of exposing fresh ways to acquire exercise without breaking up the remainder of your routine.

A lot of individuals view TV as the foe once it comes to physical action, but it doesn't have to be that way. Consider the amount of time you spend on the sofa watching television, and then consider that you're able to still watch those shows while you're on an exercise bike or treadmill.

Pick a certain show you love, and make it a "physical action show," which you only view while exercising. A lot of shows are available to purchase or rent on DVD, and hour-long programs last 45 minutes, without the commercials---the perfect length for a great workout.

Get on the bicycle or treadmill, and turn on the show. Once the closing credits come up, quit and hit the shower.

Break Binge Eating

Every time that you discover yourself thinking of what you'll have for dinner, follow that thought with what you're able to do to promote fitness. For example, you might think, 'I'd love to have a chicken dinner tonight and a bowl of raspberry sherbet. Then, I might enjoy a nice evening walk around the neighborhood.' You're letting your brain follow a mental affiliation of eating with a physical action. Remember, to achieve weight loss you have to regularly burn more calories than you consume.

If you eat right for a while, you'll distinguish that automatically things begin clicking. Your life all of a sudden becomes much greater and you see that you begin gaining control of it. And all this occurs because you've now taken control of your eating habits.

The most important thing is that you have to remain driven. Likely you started with an 'eat right' plan as you had a few extra pounds in your body. Through your constant efforts, you've now managed to defeat that situation. Your body is in much better shape now.

However that doesn't mean you're able to start going on food binges now. You have to continue with your healthy eating regimen. Only then will you feel its true effects in managing your life.

If you remain a healthy eating system for 2 months at a stretch, you'll stay on it for life. That's a fact. Therefore, it's merely those 2 months that you have to remain centered.

You'll discover that the benefits you get within those 2 months will keep you hooked onto the program forever and a day.

CHAPTER 4- HOW TO KEEP UP WITH REGULATED EATING

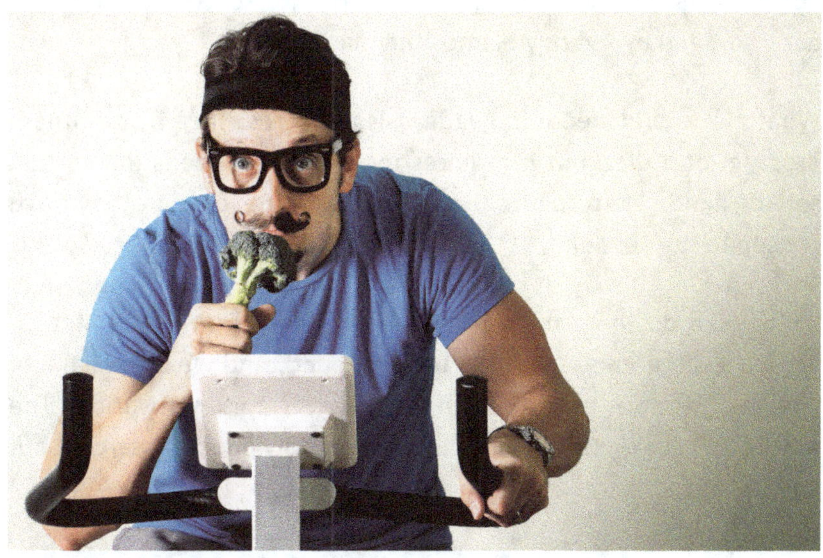

It occurs so very frequently - we resolve to go on with a health and physical fitness program with zest and likely much fanfare too; however in the first week of going into the plan, everything peters out.

Why is it that we don't stick with the diet plans, the morning jogging plans, the physical exercise plans that we make?

And what may we do to ensure we keep going with these plans, for our own sake and for the sake of the individuals that are dependent on us?

Are you eating simply to satisfy your appetite or to make your taste buds happy? Or are you eating in order to take better command of your life?

If we hear about the failure of diets or gym plans all around us, commonly it isn't their fault. Commonly it is the fault of the individuals who started with much commotion about going through these plans, telling all their acquaintances and co-workers about it, and then didn't abide by those programs. The individuals who abandon the exercise or diet halfway do not see the advantages, naturally, and everybody blames the plan.

What the world needs nowadays isn't a fresh health or fitness program or a diet, but it requires motivation. It needs the correct sort of mind-set to follow through with whatever plan they have chosen to the very end.

If they can do that, most of the health issues that are related to life- style situations will get to be outmoded. And we don't have to visit the corners of the earth to discover this motivation. The motivation lies right here, inside us; we simply need to search it out and utilize it.

One generation ago, individuals wouldn't dream of picking up whatever junk food they could get in order to feed their faces. Nowadays, we do that so very casually. "I'm hungry" commonly means "I want a burger or a hot dog, likely with chips on the side and some cola." And, "I am on a diet" means "I am on a chemically ridden pill which will defeat my hunger and deprive my body of vitamins."

It's genuinely no wonder that we are facing so many health issues today.

Our health is an indicator of what we consume. The sorry condition that we're living in isn't an individual problem; it's a global issue. The world as a whole is eating incorrectly. Six in every ten individuals in the US is overweight, and the number is going to be eight in every ten individuals by the time we hit 2015.

Are we truly thinking about this? We aren't. Even as you're studying this book, you likely have a packet of chips on the side. Do you know that what you spent on that package, which is filling your stomach with some of the most toxic chemicals known to humanity, could instead have fed an emaciated youngster in Ruanda?

But it's not simply about being philanthropic. It's about ourselves too. Yes, we have to be selfish. With such appalling health figures, aren't we heading for doom? We're definitely not eating right. Whatever excess baggage that brings - obesity and the assorted ill health in its wake - we have to be prepared for it.

So the next time you see that a program has failed or is receiving a lot of criticism, remember that the criticism isn't probably because the program stands on shaky ground. In most cases, it is because people began with great intentions and then did not follow the program as they should have.

What Matters Most

The most crucial thing that you need to keep your health and fitness program alive - even more crucial than an instructor or a doctor - is your own motive.

You have to be determined to scrutinize the situation. So, you're overweight and are looking at casting off a few pounds. No gym instructor from anyplace in the world will help you if you don't take adequate measures to have the right diet and to stick to your routine exercise.

Even if you're sick and are looking at treatment, no physician will help if you aren't determined in following the treatment platform, whether it's taking the medication at the correct time or abstaining from some foods.

We have strayed horribly with our eating habits thus far. Unless we take stock of the state of affairs and take matters in our own hands, matters are not going to get better.

The number 1 thing is awareness. We have to learn what foods are correct for us and what are not. We have to go back to training and comprehend what the nutrients are that your body truly wants and in what amount.

Then we have to build a dietary regimen for ourselves and our loved ones so that we eat healthier. We have to cut down on all the foods that are adverse - the sugars, the fats, the carbohydrates, we don't truly want them - and incorporate foods that may boost our health.

This does sound too preachy, I understand. But that's the only reprieve we have got. If we continue munching on Oreos, we're never going to get better.

But there's hope. Hope lies in the fact that there are a lot of foods out there that are simply as tasty as those awful junk foods but we don't yet know about them.

These are the foods that we don't know about yet, we likely don't care for them or as we don't know how to fix them, but a healthy cookbook may help you in understanding assorted interesting ways to healthy cooking.

Even with the same sort of diet you eat, you are able to conjure up some really delicious healthy dishes. Yes, it's all very much possible.

You are able to modify your eating habits to a big extent, while at the same time attending to your palate.

The fact is that the weight loss industry is responsible in a really significant way towards this downfall of the developed human race. They have to keep selling their Atkinses and Jenny Craigs and Zones and Medifasts and for that reason the media never tells you how we may in reality take things in your own hands.

They show us glitzy before-after pictures of a person with a foot-long sub and then the same guy with 6 pack abs and tell us that the diet made that possible.

However the fact is if we were to get our head together, we may very easily do that too, without having to spend 1000s of dollars on those diets. And what do we have to do?

2 general things:-

Control what we consume. Indulge in physical exertion.

Now, is that too much to accomplish? Don't we owe that to our body that has served us so well all these years? Don't we owe that to ourselves and our loved ones?

Why Do You Need to Eat Right?

Let's immediately plunge into the subject.

You Get Healthier

We might whole collection of books about the health advantages of eating correctly and still it wouldn't quite cover what advantages genuinely exist. The most important advantage is that you gain command over your weight.

By eating correctly, you likewise make certain that your metabolic functions - most notably your immune system and your gastrointestinal system - keep working correctly. You're likewise protected from assorted chronic diseases, right from cardiovascular diseases like coronary artery disease and high blood pressure to diabetes.

More Cost Effective

Eating healthy means you spend much less. Your bills at the supermarkets come down drastically and you don't plunge farther into charge card debt if that is already an issue with you. In addition to that, you save a huge bundle on all the healthcare expenses you'd need if any issue surfaces because of your food binging habits.

Fewer Toxins in Your Body

A lot of foods nowadays are toxic because of the synthetic chemicals present in them. When you're attempting to eat correctly, you are much less likely to get these toxins into your body as one of the basic dogmas of eating correctly is that you shouldn't eat anything that's man-made.

In addition to that, if you eat less, you'll likewise be able to reduce on vices like smoking and alcoholism. A glass of beer is almost synonymous with a night out with the boys. If you eat less, you won't want the beer as well. Similarly, you will not want that one (or more) mandatory smoke that you tend to have after each meal.

More Physical Lifestyle

When you eat better, you'll find that you are able to do your work in a much better way. You are able to exercise more, travel more, play more, work more and therefore make your life more productive.

That sure beats being a fat slob and lounging around on the couch the whole day, doesn't it? You are able to also be more involved with your friends and loved ones and that surely enriches your life.

Good Social Life

Forget about fat fetishism, individuals who are overweight don't look appealing. There's a strong social taboo about weight on the wrong places of the body. If you're trying to find a partner, your flab may literally get in the way. Not simply that, individuals who can't control their eating habits and hence their weight are looked down upon by society as being individuals who can't control their basic urges.

This sort of psychology does exist, though very few individuals will speak about it. When you eat correctly, you'll discover that such issues disappear.

Chapter 5- What is Healthy Eating?

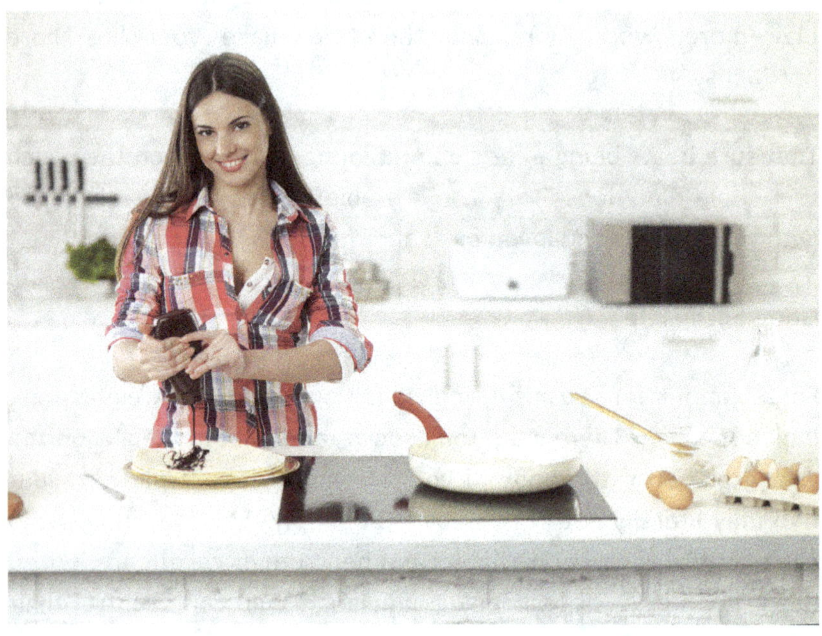

There are a lot of popular diets on the market nowadays, but most of them are unhealthy and occasionally even unsafe. This will explain how to eat a healthy, balanced diet for life and keep away from unhealthy diets.

Ascertain how many calories your body requires to function every day.

This number may vary wildly, depending on your metabolism and how physically active you are. If you're the sort of individual who puts on ten pounds simply smelling a slice of pizza, then your every day caloric intake ought to stay approximately 2000 calories for men, and 1500 calories for women.

Your body mass likewise plays a part in that: More calories are appropriate for naturally bigger individuals and fewer calories for littler individuals. If you're the sort of individual who can eat without gaining a pound, or you're physically active, you might wish to increase your daily caloric intake by 1000-2000 calories, a bit less for women.

Don't dread fatty foods.

You have to consume fat from foods for your body to run correctly. But, it's crucial to pick out the correct sorts of fats: Most animal fats and a few vegetable oils are high in the sort of fats that raise your LDL cholesterol levels; the foul cholesterol.

Different than popular belief, eating cholesterol doesn't inevitably bring up the amount of cholesterol in your body. If you provide your body the correct tools, it will flush extra cholesterol from your body. Those tools are monounsaturated fatty acids, which you ought to try to consume regularly. Foods that are rich in monounsaturated fatty acids are olive oil, nuts, fish oil, and assorted seed oils.

Eat plenty of the correct carbs.

You have to eat foods high in carbs since they're your body's chief source of energy. The trick is to pick out the correct carbs. Simple carbs like sugar and refined flour are quickly absorbed by the body's gastrointestinal system.

This induces a sort of carb overload, and your body releases vast amounts of insulin to battle the overload. Not only is the excess insulin bad on your heart, however it encourages weight gain. Eat plenty of carbs, but consume carbs that are slowly digested by the body such as whole grain flour, veggies, oats, and unprocessed grains.

Eat bigger meals early on in the day.

Your metabolism decelerates toward the end of the evening and is less efficient at digesting foods. That means more of the power stored in the food will be stacked away as fat and your body won't absorb as many nutrients from the meal. Try eating a medium-sized meal for breakfast, a big meal for lunch, and a little meal for dinner. Better yet, attempt consuming 4-6 small meals over the run of your day.

Provide yourself a cheat meal.

Cheating doesn't mean gorging on all the wrong foods once a week; it implies enjoying a food you truly love once a week. Have a couple slices of pizza on Sundays, or a huge slice of double chocolate cake on Saturdays. This cheat meal will help you stick with the change in diet, and in a few ways it's really good for your body. Special occasions, like birthdays in the family, count as cheat meals.

Get the habit of eating slowly.

It will satisfy you with fewer calories and will forestall overeating and obesity with all its consequences.

Drink plenty of H2O.

It makes you feel more awake and energized, does wonders for your skin and makes you feel fuller so you wind up eating less! Cutting down soda and replacing it with water will do wonders for you.

Keep a Record of Your Improvement

A Really crucial thing for you to do when you're on a health and wellness program is to keep checking how you're progressing. This may keep you highly motivated, particularly when you see that you're becoming what you wish yourself to become.

So, when you're on a diet program, weigh yourself frequently, doesn't matter even if you do it many times a day. When you're jogging, check how many steps you are able to climb without breathing. When you're working out at the gym, keep checking your abs and chest. When you're on a program to better your blood sugar level or your blood pressure, keep monitoring yourself. As a matter of fact, go for more frequent physical checkups just to see how well you're progressing.

Humans are very much result-oriented individuals. We wish to see facts and figures - we wish to see things as raw as they may be. This is the reason why charting your progress continuously may assist you immensely.

Once you see that your waist size has come down from 38" to 36", once you see that you are able to get into skimpier shorts, once you see that you're closer to touching your toes than before, you get very much pleased with yourself. You see that your efforts are bearing fruit. This keeps the fire ablaze.

Initially, you'll want to monitor yourself rather often. Your family might even mock you for that. But it doesn't matter. You have to know where you're heading. So keep looking as much as you wish. It is only when you're in love with your body that you'll think of doing something for it. And no one loves your body more than you, so the onus of making it fitter and healthier is totally on you.

You have every right to know how your body is progressing. The best part is that this spurs you on to do better for your body. So keep monitoring yourself and keep working out to your heart's content.

If you eat right for a while, you'll discover that automatically things begin falling into place. Your life all of a sudden becomes much better and you see that you begin gaining control of it. And all this occurs because you have now taken charge of your eating habits.

The most crucial thing is that you have to remain driven. Likely you started with an „eat right" plan as you had some extra pounds in your body. Through your constant efforts, you've now managed to defeat that situation. Your body is in much better shape now.

But that doesn't mean you are able to start going on food binges now. You have to carry on with your healthy eating regimen. Only then will you feel its true effects in managing your life.

If you remain a healthy eating program for 2 months at a stretch, you will stay on it for life. That's a fact. Therefore, it is merely those 2 months that you have to remain centered.

You'll discover that the advantages you get within those 2 months will keep you hooked onto the program forever and a day.

Chapter 6- Healthy Fitness and Healthy Food Promotes Longer Life

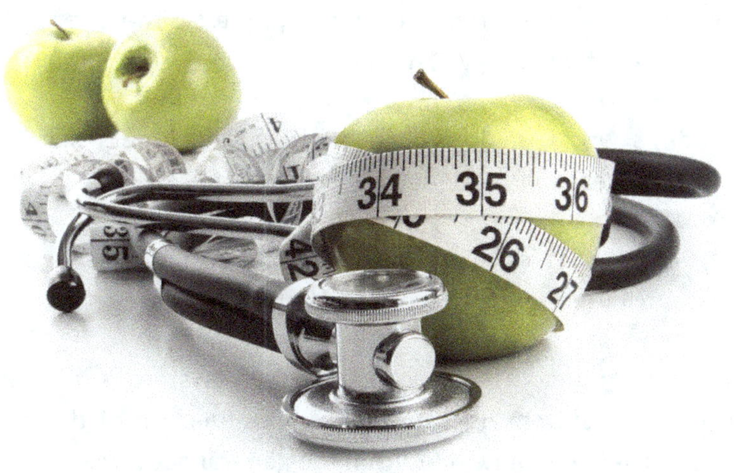

In simple terms the body has two very different and complex systems of energy producing sources. As energy is vital to the very existence of human activity and survival the two energy style depend on each other for support. This book shows you what foods give you the most energy.

It occurs so very frequently - we resolve to go on with a health and physical fitness program with zest and likely much fanfare too; however in the first week of going into the plan, everything peters out.

Why is it that we don't stick with the diet plans, the morning jogging plans, the physical exercise plans that we make?

And what may we do to ensure we keep going with these plans, for our own sake and for the sake of the individuals that are dependent on us?

Energy is needed for the various functions like maintenance of growth, daily activities, exercise and many other movements or functions that are often taken for granted. These are shared between the two energy systems.

In today's world, seldom do any health and fitness plans work. What's the reason for their alarming rate of failure?

The world is a lot less healthful than it was two decades ago. Much this is attributed to the altered food habits of individuals.

The primary and first to be used energy system is the aerobic system. This system uses oxygen for the function of the muscles and does demand quite a lot from the general body system.

This demand usually increases the rate and depth of breathing and blood supply mainly because of the corresponding increase of the heart rate.

When the body requires more energy which cannot be met due to the elevated need for more oxygen then the body system automatically switched to the anaerobic energy system. This system is able to produce energy without the need to use oxygen.

All this energy is generated through the suitable or correct consumption of foods. The foods consumed dictate the types of energy levels each individual is capable of producing.

Muscle fatigue usually occurs when all the energy sources are exhausted which can be attributed to a variety of reasons; the most compelling one depends very much on the types of foods consumed.

There are several categories of foods that produce various beneficial elements for the human body system and noting the ones that create or enhance the energy generating sources is definitely useful to know. Therefore this knowledge should help the individual choose the right types of foods.

The aerobic system works by breaking down the carbohydrates, fatty acids and amino acids in the foods consumed while the anaerobic system releases energy from the foods stored in the body, usually during intense activity bouts.

If we hear about the failure of diets or gym plans all around us, commonly it isn't their fault. Commonly it is the fault of the individuals who started with much commotion about going through these plans, telling all their acquaintances and co-workers about it, and then didn't abide by those programs.

The individuals who abandon the exercise or diet halfway do not see the advantages, naturally, and everybody blames the plan.

What the world needs nowadays isn't a fresh health or fitness program or a diet, but it requires motivation. It needs the correct sort of mind-set to follow through with whatever plan they have chosen to the very end.

If they can do that, most of the health issues that are related to life- style situations will get to be outmoded. And we don't have to visit the corners of the earth to discover this motivation. The motivation lies right here, inside us; we simply need to search it out and utilize it.

One generation ago, individuals wouldn't dream of picking up whatever junk food they could get in order to feed their faces. Nowadays, we do that so very casually. "I'm hungry" commonly means "I want a burger or a hot dog, likely with chips on the side and some cola." And, "I am on a diet" means "I am on a chemically ridden pill which will defeat my hunger and deprive my body of vitamins." It's genuinely no wonder that we are facing so many health issues today.

Our health is an indicator of what we consume. The sorry condition that we're living in isn't an individual problem; it's a global issue. The world as a whole is eating incorrectly. Six in every ten individuals in the US is overweight, and the number is going to be eight in every ten individuals by the time we hit 2015.

Are we truly thinking about this? We aren't. Even as you're studying this book, you likely have a packet of chips on the side. Do you know that what you spent on that package, which is filling your stomach with some of the most toxic chemicals known to humanity, could instead have fed an emaciated youngster in Ruanda?

But it's not simply about being philanthropic. It's about ourselves too. Yes, we have to be selfish. With such appalling health figures, aren't we heading for doom? We're definitely not eating right. Whatever excess baggage that brings - obesity and the assorted ill health in its wake - we have to be prepared for it.

So the next time you see that a program has failed or is receiving a lot of criticism, remember that the criticism isn't probably because the program stands on shaky ground. In most cases, it is because people began with great intentions and then did not follow the program as they should have.

CHAPTER 7- KNOW WHAT YOU EAT

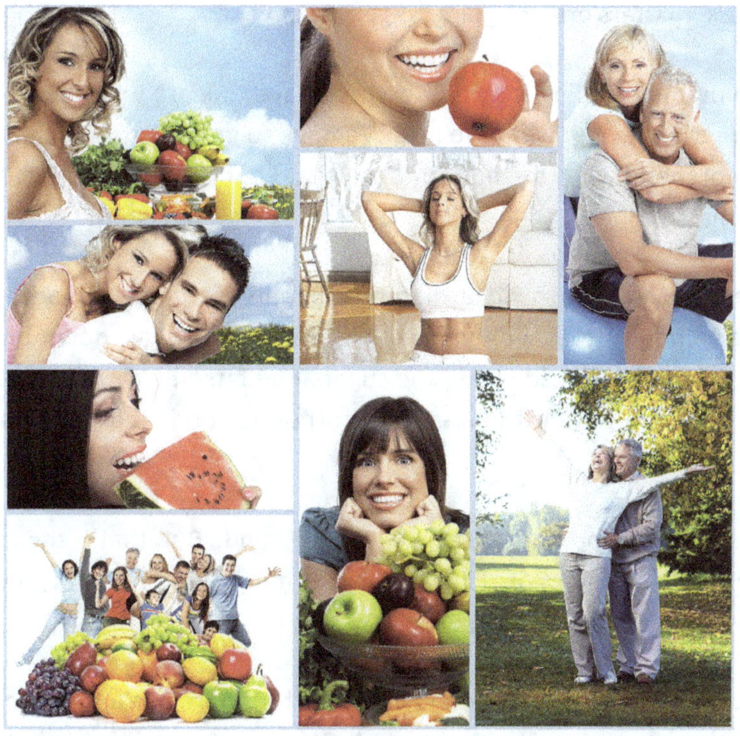

The most crucial thing that you need to keep your health and fitness program alive - even more crucial than an instructor or a doctor - is your own motive.

You have to be determined to scrutinize the situation. So, you're overweight and are looking at casting off a few pounds. No gym instructor from anyplace in the world will help you if you don't take adequate measures to have the right diet and to stick to your routine exercise.

Even if you're sick and are looking at treatment, no physician will help if you aren't determined in following the treatment platform, whether it's taking the medication at the correct time or abstaining from some foods.

Break Binge Eating
We have strayed horribly with our eating habits thus far. Unless we take stock of the state of affairs and take matters in our own hands, matters are not going to get better.

The number 1 thing is awareness. We have to learn what foods are correct for us and what are not. We have to go back to training and comprehend what the nutrients are that your body truly wants and in what amount.

Then we have to build a dietary regimen for ourselves and our loved ones so that we eat healthier. We have to cut down on all the foods that are adverse - the sugars, the fats, the carbohydrates, we don't truly want them - and incorporate foods that may boost our health.

This does sound too preachy, I understand. But that's the only reprieve we have got. If we continue munching on Oreos, we're never going to get better.

But there's hope. Hope lies in the fact that there are a lot of foods out there that are simply as tasty as those awful junk foods but we don't yet know about them.

These are the foods that we don't know about yet, we likely don't care for them or as we don't know how to fix them, but a healthy cookbook may help you in understanding assorted interesting ways to healthy cooking.

Even with the same sort of diet you eat, you are able to conjure up some really delicious healthy dishes. Yes, it's all very much possible. You are able to modify your eating habits to a big extent, while at the same time attending to your palate.

The fact is that the weight loss industry is responsible in a really significant way towards this downfall of the developed human race. They have to keep selling their Atkinses and Jenny Craigs and Zones and Medifasts and for that reason the media never tells you how we may in reality take things in your own hands.

They show us glitzy before-after pictures of a person with a foot-long sub and then the same guy with 6 pack abs and tell us that the diet made that possible.

However the fact is if we were to get our head together, we may very easily do that too, without having to spend 1000s of dollars on those diets. And what do we have to do?

2 general things:-

Control what we consume. Indulge in physical exertion.

Now, is that too much to accomplish? Don't we owe that to our body that has served us so well all these years? Don't we owe that to ourselves and our loved ones?

Honey and Whole Grains

Over the years honey has been proven to the one sustaining power behind the energy circle. Benefiting the human body in various areas it is foremost still unrivaled in its energy producing entity. Honey is nature's most natural energy booster. It also acts as an effective immunity system builder while providing the natural remedy to a host of varied ailments too.

Energy is very important to the smooth flowing natural of a daily life cycle of any human being. Therefore finding energy sources that are both consistent and healthy are important to keeping fit and happy.

The natural benefits of honey has been widely acknowledged and accepted. Besides its great taste, honey is also a natural source of carbohydrate, which is an energy maker for boosting performance, endurance and reducing levels of muscle fatigue.

This is especially useful for athletes. The sugar content in the honey helps to play a role in preventing fatigue during exercise sessions and also during training sessions for sports enthusiast. These sugar make ups are divided into glucose and fructose and functions in different but complimenting ways.

The glucose content in the honey is generally absorbed at a faster rate and gives off an immediate energy boost while the fructose works at a slower pace for a more sustainable and prolonged energy dispersement. When it comes to addressing blood sugar levels in the body system, honey has been known to help keep the levels fairly constant.

As honey is a pleasant food product and it's natural in its form, consuming it is not a very difficult exercise. People of all ages are generally quite willing to consume honey in any of its accompanying forms. It's even popular with children.

The energy produced from consuming a small amount of honey daily helps children cope with the physical strains of daily school activities and sports commitments. For the adults too consuming a daily small dose of honey can go a long way in keeping the energy levels at its best during a demanding day at work.

Making sandwiches with honey accompanied with other fillings is one way of creating a pleasant snack. Applying honey on a freshly toasted slice of bread is also a welcome breakfast alternative. Adding honey to drinks instead of using sugar is definitely encouraged.

Most people today want a quick fix for their energy boosting needs and this usually comes in the unhealthy forms of sports drinks, coffee and refined carbohydrates like sugar and while bread.

Though these produce the desired heightened energy levels, it should be noted that this energy is fairly short lived and the tiredness that follows is usually more acutely felt. Therefore opting to consume some form of whole grains is not only a better alternative but is also much healthier.

Whole grains provide the energy that comes in a more complex form which breaks down over a longer period of time. This then creates the platform for sustaining the energy levels for longer periods.

Because of its more complex make up the whole grains come with a array of beneficial elements like minerals, vitamins, phytonutrients and fiber which are also rich in fiber.

Adding the whole grain ingredients is any dish more often than not completes the flavor or enhances it altogether. Whole grains can the various forms such as wheat, oat, barley, maize, brown rice, faro, spelt, emmer, einkorn, rye, millet, buckwheat, and many more.

These can then be made into various other products like whole wheat flour, whole wheat bread, whole wheat pasta, rolled oats or oat groats, triticale flour, popcorn and teff flour.

Break Binge Eating

The benefits of consuming whole grains consistently can help decrease the risk of heart disease, lower cholesterol levels protect against many types of cancer and assist in weight management. Whole grains should not be confused with its lesser and more refined "cousin". Though refined grains have some benefits it is always better to opt for the whole grain alternatives.

CHAPTER 8- YOUR HIGH PROTEIN DIET

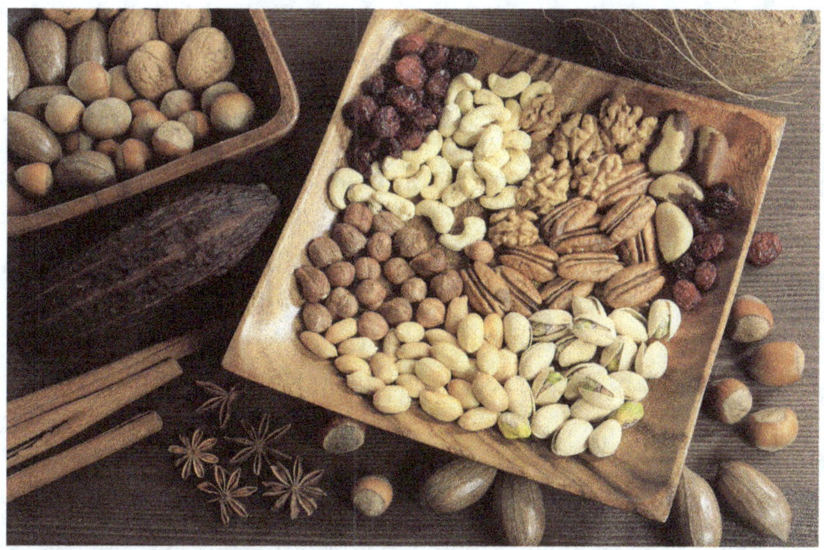

Nuts are an important source of nutrients for both human and animal consumption. Being rich in a whole host of necessary nutrients it can be eaten in its raw form, cooked or as an additive to already pre existing dishes. Thought nuts are defined as a hard shelled fruit, there are many other foods that are included in the nut family.

Different types of meats generally contribute to a variety of flavors; however the healthiest type is the one with as much lean meat content as possible. Its undisputed fact that the meats that contain a good amount of fat are a culinary treat indeed but for health purposes taking the time to understand the benefits of consuming lean meats is very wise indeed.

It is now common knowledge that nuts greatly help in keeping a lot of ailments in check or from occurring at all. For instance, nuts have been known to be able to keep the possibility of coronary heart diseases manifesting, even for those whole come from a long line of family members with this problem.

Consuming nuts like almonds and walnuts have been known to lower serum cholesterol concentrations within the body system. Nuts are also highly recommended for those individuals suffering from insulin resistance problems like diabetics.

Turning to nuts rather that junk food to quell cravings is also another healthier alternative. Containing essential fatty acids is also another plus point when it comes to choosing nuts as a healthier alternative. Because nuts are healthy and can be consumed in its raw form, it is also another added advantage to keeping these around and handy as snacks.

Almonds are often used to normalize blood lipids because of their slow burn characteristics, which help to keep the blood sugar levels consistently healthy. Rich in a varied amount of different nutrients the almond is a popular additive to the stale diet of most Mediterranean people.

The Brazil nut is also another nutritious nut which comes with its own set of benefits when consumed in moderation. Noted for its omega 3 fatty acid content, the Brazil nut is also a good source of calcium.

Cashew nut is another very popular nut that is often consumed as a salted snack. However it would be a much healthier food product without the addition of salt, as it is already quite a flavorful nut on its own. In some parts of the world these nuts are made into oils.

The selection process should be done with a little knowledge as depending solely on what the naked eye perceives is not enough. Generally lean meats derived from beef cuts should include round, chuck, sirloin and tenderloin, while the cuts from pork or lamb would constitute tenderloin, loin chops and leg. The leanest parts of the poultry would be the breast area without the skin.

Though there are many reasons people eliminate meat from their daily diet, there is no evidence to show that this is a good or bad choice not should it be followed by all.

However the important point to note here is the choice of the types of meats that would make the consumption healthy and this would generally mean meats with lesser amount of fat content. Though white meat is by no means lacking in fat content, it is by comparison much less in fat content than red meats.

The nutritional value of consuming lean meats is quite extensive and rounded. Lean meats have a generally higher and purer content of protein which is a very important contributing factor to fundamental structural and functional progress of every cell sustenance and formation.

Lean meats are also a good source of essential amino acids particularly sulphur amino acids. When compared to the digestive rates the proteins in meats work faster than the one contained in the beans and whole wheat range.

Lean meat is also a good source of iron. Because iron deficiency is progressive it is often not detected until a later stage where anemia has developed.

You Get Healthier

We might whole collection of books about the health advantages of eating correctly and still it wouldn't quite cover what advantages genuinely exist. The most important advantage is that you gain command over your weight.

By eating correctly, you likewise make certain that your metabolic functions - most notably your immune system and your gastrointestinal system - keep working correctly. You're likewise protected from assorted chronic diseases, right from cardiovascular diseases like coronary artery disease and high blood pressure to diabetes.

More Cost Effective

Eating healthy means you spend much less. Your bills at the supermarkets come down drastically and you don't plunge farther into charge card debt if that is already an issue with you. In addition to that, you save a huge bundle on all the healthcare expenses you'd need if any issue surfaces because of your food binging habits.

Less Toxins In Your Body

A lot of foods nowadays are toxic because of the synthetic chemicals present in them. When you're attempting to eat correctly, you are much less likely to get these toxins into your body as one of the basic dogmas of eating correctly is that you shouldn't eat anything that's man-made.

In addition to that, if you eat less, you'll likewise be able to reduce on vices like smoking and alcoholism. A glass of beer is almost synonymous with a night out with the boys. If you eat less, you won't want the beer as well. Similarly, you will not want that one (or more) mandatory smoke that you tend to have after each meal.

More Physical Lifestyle

When you eat better, you'll find that you are able to do your work in a much better way. You are able to exercise more, travel more, play more, work more and therefore make your life more productive.

That sure beats being a fat slob and lounging around on the couch the whole day, doesn't it? You are able to also be more involved with your friends and loved ones and that surely enriches your life.

Good Social Life

Forget about fat fetishism, individuals who are overweight don't look appealing. There's a strong social taboo about weight on the wrong places of the body. If you're trying to find a partner, your flab may literally get in the way. Not simply that, individuals who can't control their eating habits and hence their weight are looked down upon by society as being individuals who can't control their basic urges.

This sort of psychology does exist, though very few individuals will speak about it. When you eat correctly, you'll discover that such issues disappear.

There are a lot of popular diets on the market nowadays, but most of them are unhealthy and occasionally even unsafe. This will explain how to eat a healthy, balanced diet for life and keep away from unhealthy diets.

Ascertain how many calories your body requires to function every day.

This number may vary wildly, depending on your metabolism and how physically active you are. If you're the sort of individual who puts on ten pounds simply smelling a slice of pizza, then your every day caloric intake ought to stay approximately 2000 calories for men, and 1500 calories for women.

Your body mass likewise plays a part in that: More calories are appropriate for naturally bigger individuals and fewer calories for littler individuals. If you're the sort of individual who can eat without gaining a pound, or you're physically active, you might wish to increase your daily caloric intake by 1000-2000 calories, a bit less for women.

Don't dread fatty foods.

You have to consume fat from foods for your body to run correctly. But, it's crucial to pick out the correct sorts of fats: Most animal fats and a few vegetable oils are high in the sort of fats that raise your LDL cholesterol levels; the foul cholesterol.

Different than popular belief, eating cholesterol doesn't inevitably bring up the amount of cholesterol in your body. If you provide your body the correct tools, it will flush extra cholesterol from your body. Those tools are monounsaturated fatty acids, which you ought to try to consume regularly. Foods that are rich in monounsaturated fatty acids are olive oil, nuts, fish oil, and assorted seed oils.

Eat plenty of the correct carbs.

You have to eat foods high in carbs since they're your body's chief source of energy. The trick is to pick out the correct carbs. Simple carbs like sugar and refined flour are quickly absorbed by the body's gastrointestinal system.

This induces a sort of carb overload, and your body releases vast amounts of insulin to battle the overload. Not only is the excess insulin bad on your heart, however it encourages weight gain. Eat plenty of carbs, but consume carbs that are slowly digested by the body such as whole grain flour, veggies, oats, and unprocessed grains.

Eat bigger meals early on in the day.

Your metabolism decelerates toward the end of the evening and is less efficient at digesting foods. That means more of the power stored in the food will be stacked away as fat and your body won't absorb as many nutrients from the meal. Try eating a medium-sized meal for breakfast, a big meal for lunch, and a little meal for dinner. Better yet, attempt consuming 4-6 small meals over the run of your day.

Provide yourself a cheat meal.

Cheating doesn't mean gorging on all the wrong foods once a week; it implies enjoying a food you truly love once a week. Have a couple slices of pizza on Sundays, or a huge slice of double chocolate cake on Saturdays. This cheat meal will help you stick with the change in diet, and in a few ways it's really good for your body. Special occasions, like birthdays in the family, count as cheat meals.

Get the habit of eating slowly.

It will satisfy you with fewer calories and will forestall overeating and obesity with all its consequences.

Drink plenty of H2O.

It makes you feel more awake and energized, does wonders for your skin and makes you feel fuller so you wind up eating less! Cutting down soda and replacing it with water will do wonders for you.

About the Author

Frederick Morgan loves cooking. He is from a family of great cook. Great cooking and scrumptious food are not new to him. He was once obese and can't control on his eating habit. During his early twenties he can't contain all the bullying and thus, he decided to make a major transformation for his own good.

From then on, Frederick is health conscious, health buff and became a certified health instructor.